Contents

Burning Calories: Drink Ice Water 8
Burning Calories: Burn Them Fast 10
Burning Calories: Burn Them Easily 12
Burning Calories: By Spinning 14
Burning Calories: Eat Right 16
All About Working The Transverse Abdominals 18
Aquasize To A Flatter Stomach! 20
Why Do People Do Exercises For The Stomach 22
Different Exercises To Get A Flat Stomach 24
All About Free Exercises To Flatten The Stomach Fast 26
How To Target Your Stomach With Yoga 28
Lose Your Belly by Improving Your Posture 30
Six Poor Stomach Exercise Habits 32
Shrink Your Tummy! 34
Stomach Exercises For A Flatter Tummy 36
All About Stomach Flattening Exercises 38
The Post-Partum Tummy Routine 40
The Stomach Exercise All-Stars 42
The Strong Stomach Workout 44
Using Resistance Bands In Stomach Exercises 46
Burning Calories: Overview 48
Burning Calories Versus Burning Fat 50
Burning Calories: Keep Moving 52
Burning Calories: Aerobics 54
Burning Calories: Tips For Fast Burning 56
Burning Calories: Treadmills 58
Burning Calories For Weight Loss 60
Burning Calories: Track The Burning 62
Burning Calories: In Everyday Activities 64
Burning Calories Through Multi-Muscle Activities 66

Burning Calories: Drink Ice Water

For anyone trying to lose weight, this question is bound to raise a lot of excitement. Surely losing weight cannot be such a simple issue, can it? Well, the answer is YES!

You can actually lose calories by drinking ice water. Your body loses calories in the process of warming this ice water to the body temperature. Now any enthusiast, must surely be thinking, if we can lose weight by drinking ice water, can we lose a large amount of calories if we drink lots of ice water? Well, to answer this question we have to look at some simple calculations.

First of all we need to distinguish between calories and Calories. Calories (i.e. with a big c) are used to denote the amount of energy that is contained in food. Where as calorie with a small c is used to denote the energy required to raise the temperature of 1 gram of water 1 degree Celsius.

Another interesting fact is that it takes, 1 Calorie to raise the temperature of 1 kilogram of water by 1 degree Celsius. So when you are drinking a 140-Calorie can of cola, you are in fact ingesting 140,000 calories in your body. This is the same when you burn say 100 Calories working out, this means that you have actually burned 100,000 calories.

The main purpose of telling you that the definition of calories is based on the rising of temperature is to tell you an interesting fact. We have just seen that when our body raises the temperature, it burns calories, so when you drink ice cold water your body loses calories in raising that ice cold water to body temperature.

Now let us get the math right.

Our body temperature is at 37 degree Celsius.

The temperature of ice cold water can be safely said to be 0 degree Celsius.

There are 473.18 grams in 16 fluid ounces of water.

It takes 1 calorie to raise 1 gram of water by 1 degree Celsius.

So, if your body raises the temperature of 473.18 grams of water by 37 degree Celsius it burns 17508 calories.

But this is calorie with a small c. It actually denotes only 17.5 calories. You might be thinking that losing 17.5 Calories doesn't count much compared to the calories we intake.

But, you are not going to drink just one 16 once glass of water are you? Even if you stick to the recommended minimum of 8 glasses of water you will end up burning 70 Calories in a day and that too by doing practically nothing. You can also increase the water intake if you want to shed a few extra pounds.

Well, although it is definite that drinking ice cold water helps you to burn calories you should not try to replace it with exercise. You should continue with all the weight reduction methods that you already on to. You can just boost up your effort by drinking ice cold water.

Burning Calories: Burn Them Fast

Today the obesity rate has reached an alarming figure, officially 1000 people are declared obese, every single day! Well, considering our sedentary life styles it shouldn't come as a surprise. We drive where ever we have to; we sit all day at our desk and do all our work at the click of a mouse, thanks to the internet!

Given such a lifestyle, it is inevitable that we all will become obese, but there are quick and effective ways in which you can lose weight. The best way is exercise.

No, I do not mean to say that you have to sweat it out daily in the gym for hours. Even 15 minutes of exercise can help you burn ad much as 100 calories.

The first thing tat you have to do is to make an effort to move. Remember, when you were young staying indoors would seem like a punishment, but now all you want to do is to sit at home watch TV and spend endless hours surfing.

When you have free time make sure to go out, indulge in some activity, play any game that you like playing. It will not only refresh you but, you will also end up losing a lot of calories.

To burn the extra 100 calories, here are some of the things that you can try.

Cycling: cycling for even 10 minutes can help you burn 100 calories. If you have a cycle, then make sure to go out on a cycling ride with your family. You will not only have a great day with your family, but will actually be working towards attaining a great figure.

Walking: It is one of the simplest, cheapest and the most effective way of losing calories. Brisk walking for 15 minutes will help you to attain your target of losing the 100 calories. You can slowly increase the tie you spend on walking. If you do not get adequate time to go out on a morning walk, then you can try incorporating walking in the daily activities.

What I mean to say here is that you can get adown a stop before your usual stop when at work and walk the rest of the distance. Resist the temptation of taking the lift and take the stairs.

Video workout: 15 minutes of video work out four to five times a week can help you to lose calories. Just choose the video work out that you like and get started!

Skipping: Skipping ropes are extremely effective in not only losing weight, but also toning your upper body. It helps to strengthen the heart and the lungs also.

Skipping ropes are light and cheap and can be used practically anywhere. It is important that you stretch your calves muscle before and after each skipping session.

Although initially you may find it difficult t skip for 15 minutes at a stretch, but you will be amazed at how quickly your body will be able to respond to the 15 minutes skipping slot.

Burning Calories: Burn Them Easily

To lose weight you have to go on a sensible diet and exercise regularly. You have to eat right ands work out. Yes, we all know that! But exercising and sticking to a low fat diet is not considered as doing nothing! It is a big job.

But here I have for you a great trick that will help you to lose weight, doing practically nothing! Sounds too good to be true? Well read on and you will find out how simple losing weight can be. It is one of the tricks that is rarely known by any dieter or dietician. It is an absolutely safe and fool proof method of shedding the extra calories and biding them good bye forever.

You don't have to go on a killing diet, you don't have to sweat it out in the gym and neither will you be asked to take dangerous diet pills. All you have to do is to drink ice cold water!

Yes, you have read correctly, all you need to do is to drink ice cold water; this is what I call losing weight doing nothing! Let me explain to you how this works. When you drink an eight ounce cup of ice cold water your body will burn 7.69 calories to heat the water to bring it to room temperature. Amazing! Isn't it! Now let us exploit this little trick to reach our aim of weight loss.

We have just understood that we can lose approximately 8 calories by drinking an eight ounce cup of ice cold water. The minimum water requirement of water for our body is eight glasses. So we can lose 64 calories by just drinking water, just remember to have it ice cold!

If you are really motivated then you can drink a gallon of ice water daily. Gallon water is 16 cups. Drinking 16 cups of ice water will help you lose 123 calories per day. This actually amounts to 861 calories a week! And that too by doing practically nothing!

To make you feel all the more better, let me state another fact, to lose 861 calories in the conventional manner, you would have to jog for at least for two hours! Imagine, you have lost the same amount of calories without spending two hours on rigorous exercise.

Remember that it is not a compulsion that you have to drink a gallon of water in order to lose weight; you can lose weight also by drinking 8 glasses of water daily.

Burning Calories: By Spinning

Do you want to lose weight? Do you want to have great legs? And do you want to have fun while attaining these results? If your answer to the above questions is yes, then spinning is what you need. Many people after trying out, various cardio exercise and all types of exercises have unanimously come to a conclusion that spinning is the best way to lose weight and gain a great figure.

Considering how well the classes are organized this shouldn't come as a surprise. These classes are structured in such a way so as to push an individual to give his best in an encouraging and positive atmosphere.

If you want to lose weight, then there is no better option than spinning. An average of 30 minutes of spinning will help you to burn 50 calories. No other machine exercise can give you the same result. It is a challenge and a promise! Any other "low impact" machine will take at least double the time to burn 500 calories. You can also increase the amount of calories burnt depend on the intensity of your work outs. If you are really enthusiastic and want to lose weight quickly, then you can extend the time spent spinning.

There is yet another reason why spinning is the best cardio exercise. Unlike other exercises, you can stick with spinning through out the year, there is no stopping you be it rain or shine. Well, you can't say this in case of outdoor exercises, can you? I am afraid not!

Spinning has lots of health and fitness benefits. It not only helps you lose weight, but it also helps you to build muscles. In fact, spinning is regarded as the most beneficial exercise by most of the fitness trainers.

Spinning pushes the body to the optimum level, on a personal note, after spinning I feel great! I feel as if my body has done something that I earlier thought was an impossible feat to accomplish.

Although spinning pushes he limits for the body, yet it is easy for beginners too. In fact as there is no impact of nature, so your knee and legs won't hurt. Spinning is completely safe for people of all age groups. Even older people with joint problems can easily do spinning.

Burning Calories: Eat Right

There are two simple ways in which you can lose weight. You can either lose weight by in taking fewer calories, or you can shed a few pounds by brining calories. If you want to lose weight, then cutting calories, makes a lot of sense.

But, it is important that you cut calories sensibly, because cutting too many calories, will do more harm than good. It will not only hamper your health, but it can also act as a road block to shedding weight.

Generally people have a wrong notion, that as consuming fewer calories helps to shed weight, so consuming absolutely minimal calories will help them lose faster. This is in fact, sadly untrue. Everything has to be done in moderation.

An extremely low calorie diet will not only cause harm to your body, but will also hinder your weight loss. You don't want that, do you?

When you cut down calories too low, your body interprets that you have gone in to a starvation mode.

Thus it will try its best to maintain your current weight. Your body will slow down its metabolism and so that it can save energy and store it to the fat reserve that you already have. This in fact will make it all the more difficult to lose weight.

Thus you can clearly see why cutting down calories, does the opposite of what you want it do.

Not only do these low calorie starvation diets reduce your metabolism. These are also are very harmful for the body. These causes dizziness, light headiness and you will find difficult to concentrate.

These starvation diets are also very difficult to stick to, when you feel hungry; chances are that you will not be able to resist the temptation. The end result will be that you end up gorging up food. In most cases, Starvation diets will help you to gain weight instead of losing them.

A more sensible way to lose weight is to eat right rather than not eat at all. When you feel hungry, it is important that you eat; your body should not feel that you are starving.

Eating does not mean that you can eat food dripping with oil, or gorge on snacks loaded with cheese. Instead having a glass of fruit juice or a low calorie snack should do the trick.

If you feel the need to binge, then make sure you eat light on the successive days, this way you can balance the calorie intake.

So if you want to shed weight, the simple trick is to eat! Eat, but eat right!

All About Working The Transverse Abdominals

When you are exercising it is essential that you focus on a significant muscle group which is often neglected called the transverse abdominals. These are the central muscles and they are often neglected by accident as much as by design.

Most stomach exercises focus on the vertical abs - the six-pack which you so often see in TV ads and in magazines - and with the focus on these it is perhaps not surprising. Even crunches, the most popular of abdominal exercises, do little for the transverse abdominals. But, these muscles are among the most important and should be targeted. They provide support to all areas of your torso including to your lower-back muscles. Any exercise routine with an aim of flattening or shaping the stomach should focus on these important muscles.

The following exercises will assist with developing a more complete abdominal workout and assist with that flat tummy we all crave. As with all exercise routines ensure you warm up properly before starting on these exercises;

The Pelvic Tilt
Lie on a flat surface such as a bench or the floor using a mat or a towel to cushion yourself. Bend you knees until your feet are flat on the floor. Keeping your upper body on the floor throughout slowly and with a controlled movement raise your hips from the floor. Hold it at that position for a few seconds at the top of the arc and then lower it slowly maintaining control throughout. It is important that you do not allow your body to drop suddenly while lowering as you will not be using your muscles adequately if you do. You should do a full set of these.

The Crunchless Crunch
This exercise sounds easy but can be difficult to do well. It uses different muscles to those normally used and can be tough to get right at first. Essentially in involves contracting your stomach muscles to pull your belly button back towards your spine, compressing your stomach as you do so. You can either try this lying on your back or in a kneeling position. To start relax your body. Then slowly contract your stomach as if you are pulling your belly button backwards. Hold this for ten seconds then release slowly. Once you find ten seconds easy repeat it for longer. Building this up over time will lead to a strengthening and tightening of the transverse abdominals.

A more sensible way to lose weight is to eat right rather than not eat at all. When you feel hungry, it is important that you eat; your body should not feel that you are starving.

Eating does not mean that you can eat food dripping with oil, or gorge on snacks loaded with cheese. Instead having a glass of fruit juice or a low calorie snack should do the trick.

If you feel the need to binge, then make sure you eat light on the successive days, this way you can balance the calorie intake.

So if you want to shed weight, the simple trick is to eat! Eat, but eat right!

All About Working The Transverse Abdominals

When you are exercising it is essential that you focus on a significant muscle group which is often neglected called the transverse abdominals. These are the central muscles and they are often neglected by accident as much as by design.

Most stomach exercises focus on the vertical abs - the six-pack which you so often see in TV ads and in magazines - and with the focus on these it is perhaps not surprising. Even crunches, the most popular of abdominal exercises, do little for the transverse abdominals. But, these muscles are among the most important and should be targeted. They provide support to all areas of your torso including to your lower-back muscles. Any exercise routine with an aim of flattening or shaping the stomach should focus on these important muscles.

The following exercises will assist with developing a more complete abdominal workout and assist with that flat tummy we all crave. As with all exercise routines ensure you warm up properly before starting on these exercises;

The Pelvic Tilt
Lie on a flat surface such as a bench or the floor using a mat or a towel to cushion yourself. Bend you knees until your feet are flat on the floor. Keeping your upper body on the floor throughout slowly and with a controlled movement raise your hips from the floor. Hold it at that position for a few seconds at the top of the arc and then lower it slowly maintaining control throughout. It is important that you do not allow your body to drop suddenly while lowering as you will not be using your muscles adequately if you do. You should do a full set of these.

The Crunchless Crunch
This exercise sounds easy but can be difficult to do well. It uses different muscles to those normally used and can be tough to get right at first. Essentially in involves contracting your stomach muscles to pull your belly button back towards your spine, compressing your stomach as you do so. You can either try this lying on your back or in a kneeling position. To start relax your body. Then slowly contract your stomach as if you are pulling your belly button backwards. Hold this for ten seconds then release slowly. Once you find ten seconds easy repeat it for longer. Building this up over time will lead to a strengthening and tightening of the transverse abdominals.

Scissor Kick

Again, lie on the floor, upper body and back tight to the ground. Place your hands under your buttocks to raise you slightly from the floor keeping your back pressed down flat. Slowly raise one leg to around ten inches then slowly (and I mean slowly) lower it to the floor. As you lower one leg slowly raise the other so for a short time both are in a crossing movement. Repeat the exercise for a complete set. using a slow, well-controlled speed throughout is essential and will increase the effectiveness of the exercise.

These are by no means the only exercises targeting these muscles, the transverse abdominals, but they should get you started. Stomach exercises such as this are important to any tummy-flattening plan and are especially effective for pregnant and women just after pregnancy.

Aquasize To A Flatter Stomach!

Swimming is great exercise however and whenever you do it. But as well as using the water for fun and relaxation you can use your time in the pool to help you in that search for a flatter stomach.

More so than air, water provides great natural resistance. Moving through it takes effort and can exercise your muscles more fully but more safely than many other types of exercise. It offers a low-impact way of exercising making it better for your joints and the exercise of choice for many age groups.

Try these exercises the next time you are in the pool and see what we mean. Remember to consult a medical professional before starting any new exercise routine, and make sure that you do warm up properly;

The Dig and Jump
This involves two movements, one targeted at your lower body and the other at the upper. Begin by standing in water of a depth above your navel and your chest. Then place your feet at least shoulder width apart and jump so that your knees come to the pool's surface then force them back down again and repeat the moves (picture a frog jumping while you are doing it and you'll get the idea). This is great for exercising the lower body and this includes the abdominal muscles.

The second part is to work the upper body. To start make a separate scoop with each hand. Place your hands low in the water then bring them to the surface and out to one side. Start by doing one hand first for three minutes then the other. Work alternate sides to maintain a balanced workout. Once you are comfortable with it do both hands at the same time to exercise the entire stomach region at once.

Set realistic targets as you work towards your health and fitness goals. Don't over exert yourself leading to injury. Start slow, know your limitations and build on them incrementally. As you increase endurance and strength you can vary the speed and length of the workout, and even add water gloves to increase resistance. It is important however not to compromise on the style of movement in order to increase reps or speed. It's better to do something well rather than quickly.

A few additional tips for exercising your midriff

First, a balanced diet is essential to any fitness regime. It's no use working hard only to undo all of the great work with a poor diet.

Secondly, stay hydrated not only when exercising but in your general daily life. A good rule of thumb is to take your body weight in pounds, divide it by 2 and aim to drink that number of Ounces of water per day. This will maintain a healthy balance.

Third, get enough rest. Get plenty of sleep but also the right kind of sleep. Sleeping on your stomach for example may make it difficult to do certain types of stomach exercise. Try to sleep in a number of positions. Also, it may sound strange to say so but take adequate rest from exercise. Be sure to schedule in rest days to any training schedule. Your body needs to recover so your muscles can rebuild.

By following this you will already be on the way to a toned, flat stomach.

Why Do People Do Exercises For The Stomach

Stomach exercises are certainly in vogue and most exercise routines place an emphasis on abdominal exercises. Crunches and other abdominal exercises are one of the mainstays of training programs and always have been. But why should that be the case?

There are a number of reasons. The obvious one is because of health concerns. It is a well documented fact that carrying around extra weight around your stomach areas can lead you to face more health problems. They can be at greater risk of certain medical conditions than those who are more toned. This reason alone should be enough to encourage you to exercise your stomach and abdominal muscles. This is certainly a salient reason for doctors recommending stomach exercises.

A second, related reason is that by exercising and maintaining a strong stomach area you affect all areas of your body. The stomach is the centre of your body, and a strong stomach generally means a stronger back and it makes the rest of your body more able to cope with the demands placed upon it. Most people want to feel strong whether it is so they can work better, enjoy their children or just feel better about themselves. A well-managed abdominal routine can help them to maintain this.

But often the most important factor is because of media and peer pressure to look good. A well developed set of abdominal muscles lives up to the media's idea of a good-looking body. They always talk about 'movie-star good looks' and a toned stomach is surely part of that. Not many people want to be seen with a bulging stomach overhanging their waistband. Why do you think it is that when we look at ourselves in the mirror we draw in our stomach to see how we could look? Why is it a natural reaction to suck in our stomachs when we walk past anyone we want to impress?

Recently-pregnant women tend to focus on toning up their stomachs as soon as they can after childbirth. The number of celebrity mums who get back into shape mere weeks after giving birth is part of the reason why women strive to do the same, but there is also a health boon by doing so. Strengthening their stomach muscles helps their whole body to recover from the rigors of childbirth.

Specific events also provide a driving reason to exercise and achieve a flatter, more flattering stomach. Maybe you need to get into that wedding dress (or if you are the bridesmaid maybe to look better than the bride!), or get out of your old 1-piece swimsuit into a bikini now that summer is approaching. Maybe you have a school reunion coming up and want to show that you still have it! Maybe a doctor has suggested you could do with a tune-up, or maybe its all about improving your self confidence. Whatever the reason they are all legitimate.

So although health and good looks are the two main reasons for the emphasis on stomach workouts these cover a multitude of personal reasons. Whatever the reason, as long as you are motivated to continue your program until you see results then the reason is a good one.

Different Exercises To Get A Flat Stomach

Flat stomachs do not need to be a pipe dream. Everyone can achieve what they want regardless of their financial situation, location or background. But, it will take motivation, dedication and time.

Exercising your stomach muscles can be achieved in a number of ways, some of them employing expensive equipment, others using what is to hand such as a floor and mat or a medicine ball. Certain stomach muscle groups will be exercised as part of other routines. Pilates, while providing an all round aid to fitness will have an impact on all areas of your body including the stomach, legs and back. But it tends to be the basic, focused exercises, regardless of how you do them that have the greatest impact.

The Crunch is the basis of a successful stomach routine. Crunches are a better way to exercise the body than routine sit ups as they don't put anywhere near as much strain on the back. A crunch is achieved by compressing your stomach muscles, most often by lying down and raising your upper torso a few inches from the ground. You do not need a long, excessive movement rather a short lift repeatedly used will apply pressure to the stomach muscles just where needed and the results are better.

A variation of this is the side crunch. The same basic principle applies, but the twisting motion as the crunch is completed will work the 'love handles' or obliques as they are more properly known.

The key is to make sure that your stomach muscles, not your legs, or head or arms do the work. Maintaining a straight back, shoulder and head line is important to ensure it is the stomach that is worked, and there are numerous resources across the internet that can assist you with style and methods.

As well as focusing only on the middle section of the stomach it is important that you include a range of different exercises to work all areas of the abdomen. This should pay attention to the upper and lower, side and central areas of your stomach. It will do a person no good to only focus on one specific muscle group.

Specific events also provide a driving reason to exercise and achieve a flatter, more flattering stomach. Maybe you need to get into that wedding dress (or if you are the bridesmaid maybe to look better than the bride!), or get out of your old 1-piece swimsuit into a bikini now that summer is approaching. Maybe you have a school reunion coming up and want to show that you still have it! Maybe a doctor has suggested you could do with a tune-up, or maybe its all about improving your self confidence. Whatever the reason they are all legitimate.

So although health and good looks are the two main reasons for the emphasis on stomach workouts these cover a multitude of personal reasons. Whatever the reason, as long as you are motivated to continue your program until you see results then the reason is a good one.

Different Exercises To Get A Flat Stomach

Flat stomachs do not need to be a pipe dream. Everyone can achieve what they want regardless of their financial situation, location or background. But, it will take motivation, dedication and time.

Exercising your stomach muscles can be achieved in a number of ways, some of them employing expensive equipment, others using what is to hand such as a floor and mat or a medicine ball. Certain stomach muscle groups will be exercised as part of other routines. Pilates, while providing an all round aid to fitness will have an impact on all areas of your body including the stomach, legs and back. But it tends to be the basic, focused exercises, regardless of how you do them that have the greatest impact.

The Crunch is the basis of a successful stomach routine. Crunches are a better way to exercise the body than routine sit ups as they don't put anywhere near as much strain on the back. A crunch is achieved by compressing your stomach muscles, most often by lying down and raising your upper torso a few inches from the ground. You do not need a long, excessive movement rather a short lift repeatedly used will apply pressure to the stomach muscles just where needed and the results are better.

A variation of this is the side crunch. The same basic principle applies, but the twisting motion as the crunch is completed will work the 'love handles' or obliques as they are more properly known.

The key is to make sure that your stomach muscles, not your legs, or head or arms do the work. Maintaining a straight back, shoulder and head line is important to ensure it is the stomach that is worked, and there are numerous resources across the internet that can assist you with style and methods.

As well as focusing only on the middle section of the stomach it is important that you include a range of different exercises to work all areas of the abdomen. This should pay attention to the upper and lower, side and central areas of your stomach. It will do a person no good to only focus on one specific muscle group.

As with exercise in general there are a wealth of resources available in book stores, libraries, on video and on the internet to assist with producing a balanced program. With so many options it is not unusual for people to struggle to identify the quality information from the rest. Putting a balanced stomach exercise program together is important and tailoring this to yourself is key. What suits one person will not always suit another. A person who exercises a lot will need a more demanding program than a novice, an overweight person a different one to a slim one.

While some exercises will work better for some, no exercise will work if it is not implemented properly, done well and performed frequently. A person should decide which exercise they are capable of as well as determining how long each session of training should be. They need to achieve a balance between different types of exercise. If the exercise is too complicated, takes too much time or needs specialist equipment is less likely to be successful.

Only over an extended period of time can you hope to achieve a flat stomach irrespective of the types of exercise used.

All About Free Exercises To Flatten The Stomach Fast

It is a common misconception by people seeking to change their physique that a toned, flatter stomach is going to cost them a lot. They may well gave a goal - a very specific aim - but be put off from achieving this because of these concerns. But the path to a more shapely, flatter stomach does not need to be littered with expensive equipment, costly gym memberships and hundreds of hours of dedicated time.

While making use of a gym certainly does help many people it is not the case that there are no other alternatives. Some individuals would prefer to train alone, un watched and unsupervised. While you need to make sure that what you do is safe and meaningful there is absolutely nothing wrong with that. A gym in fact may hinder your progress if you become self-conscious as a result.

Regardless of the equipment at hand, attending a gym will not guarantee results. For many, the equipment is a distraction. Instead, there are many places where you can find free advice and information on achieving a flatter more attractive stomach without a huge financial outlay.

Among some of the more common sources of information are libraries, book stores and increasingly the internet. You can find numerous free of charge illustrated, step-by-step guides on undertaking health and fitness routines including stomach exercises. There are videos for streaming or purchase from a range of sources for all sorts of different levels. Increasingly libraries have video resources for loan and by piecing the various elements together you can devise a strong, useful program that suits your needs and meets your budget.

Even without doing a lot of research there are some exercises that most people will be aware of. the most common of these is the crunch. This is a basic exercise designed to work the stomach muscles and flatten and tone the stomach muscles. There are variations in how you might implement these (and a lot of resources to show this also), but it is a simple exercise, requiring no equipment which can be very effective.

So how much money a person spends does not necessarily equate to the level of improvement a person will receive. It is of course possible that if you do invest a lot of money you may find that you are more motivated, but there's no guarantee that this is the case. But even if you do not invest a lot on gym memberships or equipment there is no reason to believe that a flat stomach is unachievable.

Exercise is not about the money you spend. So don't believe the hype. You can achieve a honed, toned body without huge financial outlay. You need dedication and a moderate investment of time. Your diet needs to be balanced and healthy. So achieving a flat stomach is within everyone's reach. It's easier than you might think.

How To Target Your Stomach With Yoga

Yoga is an excellent component of any health and fitness routine. It helps to reduce stress, aid mobility and exercise al parts of the body. And, you can use yoga in such a way as to target certain parts of the body including your stomach.

There are numerous yoga positions which can be used to exercise your stomach muscles. Called Asanas, these exercises come in varying degrees of difficulty. It is important to assess your skill and fitness levels and chose Asanas which you are comfortable with. Start with one which seems easy and work up to the more complex over a period of time. Do not be led to take on more than you are comfortable with. Be sure to seek medical advice before undertaking any new course of exercise and make sure that you warm up to avoid injury.

Some of the Asanas to improve stomach tone;

Pavan-Muktasan
First lie on your back ideally on a yoga mat or towel to protect your spine. When first starting yoga, this exercise can be completed one leg at a time. Bend your knees to your chest so your thighs touch your abdomen. Hug your knees, using one hand to hold the other. Lift your head so that your nose touches your knees then take a deep breath and hold this for thirty seconds. Release your legs and slowly lower to the starting position.

Bhujangasan
For this exercise, lie on the floor and roll onto your stomach. Place your hands under each shoulder as if to do a push up. Using only your back muscles, lift your upper torso from the ground so that your head becomes upright. You need the muscles from your back to do all the work so do not help with your hands. Although predominantly making use of your back muscles, this asana will help with developing better muscle tone in your stomach.

The Bow
This is a more advanced asana. The stomach exercise is similar in many ways to the Bhujangasan asana, but is more difficult. It starts from the same basic position - flat on your stomach - but now you also curl your legs upwards in addition to lifting your upper body. In a perfect example the soles of your feet come toward the back of your head forming a circle.

Once you can, grab your ankles, pull with your hands, push using your legs till only your stomach touches the floor. Hold this for at least thirty seconds before releasing and returning to the starting position.

Paad-Pashchimottanasan

This asana is also more advanced. Start lying on your back, relaxed with your legs straight, arms extended over your head. Point your palms to the ceiling. Using only your stomach muscles sit up, keeping your back straight and hands overhead. Your legs stay fixed to the floor throughout. Lean forward so your head is between your arms and grab your toes with both hands. Hold for 2 minutes before releasing and slowly returning to your starting position using your stomach muscles to lower yourself to the floor.

Yoga like every other form of exercise or wellness routine will be more effective when combined with a balanced diet and healthy lifestyle.

Lose Your Belly by Improving Your Posture

It sounds easy to say but your posture determines other people's perceptions of you. 'Don't slouch'. I must have heard it a thousand times as a kid but it wasn't until later in life that I realized just how important those words were. And what is important is not just standing up straight, but how each part of the body relates to others.

I'm sure that most people know the kid's song where the shoulder bone is connected to your back bone, but how many of us really take the message to heart? Of course we know that as far as the skeleton goes it's accurate; but that really isn't the point. A human body is a set of interrelated components and a change in one part of the body will affect others. So it makes sense that your posture will affect the way that your stomach appears, and the underlying strength in your muscles will naturally affect the way that you stand.

Stand up and sit up straight!
So the initial step to improving the way your stomach looks is to stand and sit straight. This stretches your back muscles and lengthens your stomach lines but it also has other effects. A decent posture will strengthen your back, strengthen your 'girdle' - the circle of muscles around your midriff - and improve your health. Just sitting and standing up straighter strengthens your abdominal muscles giving a firmer, more toned appearance. And lastly, a decent posture makes it more likely that the blood flow, to all parts of your body including your legs and back - each of which are integral to many abdominal and stomach exercises - and can add years to your life.

Back Extension
Done properly even a moderate amount of exercise can improve your posture, and completing back extensions is an ideal way to achieve this. To start this you need to lie on the floor face down, ideally on a mat or a towel. With arms by your side palms up use your back muscles to lift your upper body from the floor until your back is arched. Hold the contraction briefly then release and slowly lower your upper body back to the floor. Repeat this as a full set.

Then, still lying on the floor but face up this time straighten your arms above your head until they are fully extended. Then using your stomach and back muscles lift both legs off the floor at the same time. Hold your legs a few inches from the floor for a few seconds then lower them slowly.

Carrying out these two exercises will help you to strengthen your back muscles, enhance your abdominal muscles and straighten your posture. They are excellent simple steps to help rid yourself of an unwanted belly.

As with all exercise routines make sure that you consult a medical professional before you begin and always stretch and warm up fully to avoid injury.

Six Poor Stomach Exercise Habits

Stomach exercises can be carried out in a number of ways, but if you do them poorly not only will they not do any good, they could cause a lot of harm. When about to start an exercise program of any kind you should seek advice from a professional, and each time you should include a warm-up routine.

Specifically with stomach exercises you should remember these following points;

Keep Knees Up

Even though deep down you know you need to put in the effort, it's all too easy to cheat. Whenever you are doing any type of crunches you should have keep your feet flat to the floor, knees pointed upwards as central as possible. This does make your crunches harder to do, but the results will be better as well. More importantly, if you do move your knees to either side it can compress your spine and this can lead to painful back injuries.

Sit-ups

No matter how widely they are used, traditional sit-ups do little to improve abdominal muscles, but the scope for them doing harm is immense. Even when done properly they do not exercise the abs, rather the hip muscles. Further, when people do sit ups they tend to do them quickly and the momentum rather than the technique is what takes over so no muscle groups are worked properly. The crunch, with its shorter movement is a better alternative.

Straight Leg Lift

Traditionally put into training plans by inexperienced people, this exercise actually puts pressure on the lower back rather than working any legitimate muscle group. Often, this leads to injury rather than achieving anything meaningful.

Too Many Reps

Over-exercising on stomach exercises is a big cause of problems. You should never do more than fifty repetitions of any stomach exercise. If fifty reps is not enough you should try a more difficult exercise rather than increasing the number of reps.

Sleeping

Your sleeping position will have a significant impact on your ability to do and success at stomach exercises. Sleeping on your front can cause nagging back ache and pain, and the easiest way to make sure that you avoid that is to sleep on your back with a rolled mat or a pillow under your knees. This keeps your vertebrae in alignment, prevents back pain and allows you to work out pain free.

Low-Resistance Workouts

All exercises, but particularly stomach ones need resistance if they are to be effective. This resistance can come from resistance bands, from exercise balls or from your own body weight and gravity. Exercises which do not employ any resistance will not improve your muscle-tone or abs. Low resistance exercise does not cause any problems and can be used as an excellent warm up. But don't rely on this and expect that alone to flatten your stomachs.

Proper technique for whatever the exercises are is important. And these are only a few targeted tips to allow you to avoid wasting time and causing injuries to yourself. Be sure that you research your options thoroughly before you begin any new exercise regime, and always consult a physician or a professional before starting any physical exercise fitness routine.

Shrink Your Tummy!

The midriff is the one area which most people focus on as being their most significant health problem area. The ways that they choose to address it are varied, involving exercise, food and more drastic measures such as surgery. Except in exceptional circumstances, surgery should never be required.

A well-balanced calorific intake is one of the main tenets of a healthy, well-developed stomach, but that alone is not enough. Exercise is a key to creating the shape you want to maintain and there are numerous well-thought-out exercises to assist you.

The following exercises are designed to assist you to improve the appearance of and decrease your stomach size and the proportion of belly-fat you carry. These exercises have been created for beginners so all of you should be able to try these, but progress to a more challenging set of exercises when ready. When conducting abdominal exercises remember to do them slowly. Maintain control and do not allow the momentum of your body to take over. Just as with any exercise workout make sure you consult a medical professional before starting and ensure you warm up fully to prevent injury.

Vertical Leg Crunches

These are a variation of the more traditional crunches, but focus on reducing the amount of stomach fat. Prepare your exercise location, ideally an exercise mat or a towel on the floor or a flat bench. Then lie flat on the mat. Place both hands clasped behind your head, both elbows far enough out to the sides that they are out of sight. Then lift your legs into the air until they are straight up, crossed at the ankles and with knees slightly bent. Then, contract your abs, lift your head, upper back and shoulders to around a 30 degree angle. Try not to bend your back as this would defeat the object.

Long Arm Crunches

For these remain lying with your back flat to the floor, knees bent, feet flat. Recline back and extend both arms above your head as though reaching away from you. Contract your abdominal muscles then slowly lift both arms, your head and shoulders from the floor aiming for about 30 degrees. Hold it for a few seconds then slowly, under full control lower your back and shoulders to the floor then repeat this for a full set.

Reverse Crunches

You need to remain on your back for this abdominal exercise. Put both arms at your side, palms up. Raise your legs in the air so they are straight up, your hips make about a ninety degree angle with your torso. Now, contract your abdominal muscles so it feels like your navel is being pulled toward your spine, while at the same time gently lifting your hips off the floor. Raise your hips a few inches from the floor, keeping both legs extended upward. Hold this position, then slowly lower your hips back to the floor. Repeat this for a full set.

Stomach Exercises For A Flatter Tummy

So it's that time of year again. The weather is picking up and it won't be long before it's time to break out the bikinis and shorts. But, there's still the problem of that unsightly bulge around the waist that's been developing since Thanksgiving.

The following exercises can assist you to shed those extra pounds and flatten your stomach ready for the beach. As with all workout routines, make sure you consult with a medical professional before starting and always complete a proper warm up to prevent injury.

The Plank
For these stomach exercises you start by lying on your stomach on the floor or another flat surface. We'd recommend using a mat or a thick towel to protect your knees and hips. Rest your upper body on your forearms. Your elbows should be at about a 90 degree angle, positioned underneath your shoulders. Using your torso muscles lift your body until you are supported only by your toes and elbows. make sure that your body remains rigid, hence the name of the board. Hold the position for at least twenty seconds. This should exercise your muscles enough that you shouldn't need to do repeat reps.

The Side Plank
A variation of the Plank, you begin this in the same position as the original. Once lying flat on your stomach, roll onto your left side keeping your body supported by your left forearm. Your hips should be aligned, your right foot on top of the left, your body raised from the floor. As with the Plank you should remain rigid but this time on your side. Hold this plank position steady for five seconds then lower yourself slowly and repeat on the other side.

The Ball Roll
From the article title you might have surmised that you need a ball to complete this abdominal exercise...you don't. In this exercise you become the ball!

To start, sit on a firm surface and hug your knees bringing them to your chest. Then rock back gently so that you are balanced on your butt and tail bone with your feet held off the floor. Keep your toes pointed downwards as this stretches muscles far better. Contract your abdominal muscles in while rocking onto your lower back. Once you have settled, contract your ab muscles again and haul yourself using these muscles to your starting position. If you initially find this difficult you may choose to loosen your arms slightly to assist you.

Standing Crossover

As the name suggests this is a standing exercise but one sit can help to exercise the transverse abdominals well. Position your feet just a few inches apart then put your arms out to each side and bend your elbows so that your fingertips are pointing to the ceiling and your palms are facing forward. Tense your abs and lift your right knee to your left elbow, while at the same time bringing your left elbow down to your right knee. The cross-over movement will be very effective at exercising your abs. Touch your elbow to your knee, pause, and then return to the starting position. Switch sides and repeat this for an entire set.

All About Stomach Flattening Exercises

Pick up just about any magazine on health or fitness and there are guaranteed to be articles on stomach-firming exercises. And it is not really surprising since this is the one stand-out thing that people want - flatter, wash-board stomachs.

Some of the questions these magazines try to answer are why certain people have flatter tummies then others, and how they achieved this. looking at each in turn we can see that the reasons are numerous, but that there are common themes;

Diet
Those who are able to achieve flatter, more toned stomachs tend to eat balanced diets, with plenty of fresh fruit and vegetables, plenty of fibre and everything in moderation. If your calorific intake is significantly more than others is it any wonder that they find it easier than you?

Exercise
Some individuals spend time daily doing abdominal-flattening exercises, whilst others do not. Even if you eat well and eat healthily this is not enough to guarantee a flatter stomach.

Heredity
It is true that some people are genetically predisposed to have a certain shape. That is not to say that you cannot overcome such genetic conditioning, but it may make it easier or harder to achieve that flatter stomach you seek. Working harder, paying closer attention to your diet, exercise and conditioning will help even if you feel you are fighting an uphill battle.

Medical Conditions
Some people will find it more difficult to undertake a stomach-flattening course of exercise. Pregnant or post-partum women should take things in moderation increasing their intensity only when safe to do so, and it is essential that they do so under medical advice. Other medical conditions (skeletal, muscular and others) will also have an impact and any training plan should match their needs.

So How Can I Achieve A Firmer Stomach?

Well it is beyond question that regardless of what you have highlighted above, a training plan built around stomach firming exercises will get you the required results more quickly. Managed well, these can also counteract the problems of heredity and medical limitations.

As you probably realize there are literally hundreds of different exercises you could use, but not all are suitable for all ages, shapes and fitness levels. The Internet is a handy source of information, as are libraries, book stores and even fitness instructors. But before you start it is good to keep in mind that there are differences between flattening your stomach and building abdominal muscles, even though the methods for each can be similar.

One thing to keep in mind as a person works on stomach flattening exercise is that the routine he or she does should include exercises that are meant to flatten each different area of the stomach, and not just concentrate on one set of muscles. You will therefore need to employ a range of different exercises to be successful in flattening the stomach.

A flatter tummy can lead to more confidence, improved health and better overall strength. It is a reasonable aim to want to have a flatter stomach, but is not out of reach unless a specific medical reason exists. Remember that a flatter stomachs do not appear overnight, it takes time, energy and dedication, but the results are worth it.

The Post-Partum Tummy Routine

The joy of a new baby is a wonderful, beautiful, exciting thing. The after-effects of childbirth however can stay with a woman for a long time, and post-partum blues is often influenced by how you react to that baby belly that you will inevitably be left with.

The most effective way to set about tackling the loss of shape is to focus on a decent diet, decent exercise routine and a balance between the two. With a new baby around it might not be easy to dedicate the time you would like to getting back in shape, and the shock at having to be a stay-at-home mum with the loss of freedom that implies can't always be easy. The positive side is that exercising and eliminating extra stomach fat need not take up as much time as you might think, and it will give you additional energy. Once you get the hang of it you can actually spend quality time with your new bundle of joy.

Here are some simple exercises to help you improve your tummy;

Progressive Crunchless Crunches

This simple, low impact exercise works your stomach almost as effectively as a traditional crunch, but without straining yourself. Begin sitting comfortably on a chair. Take a deep breath, and fully expand your abdomen, then exhale in small staggered breaths as you draw your tummy in (imagine your navel being pulled toward your spine). Then contract your muscles 5 times and do a complete set of reps. You can also do this lying flat on your back. I'd suggest you try both ways and see which helps you to feel the contractions better.

Contractions

Start in the same position as a progressive crunchless crunch by taking a deep breath. Instead of pulling your tummy all the way in, exhale and pull it just halfway. Then use your abdominal muscles to pull your navel towards your spine. Contract your muscles and hold for a count of one. Repeat this from the exhalation point then do the whole thing one hundred times. The speed and repetition is what will achieve the desired results.

The Stomach Exercise All-Stars

Information overload is certainly a growing problem, and when seeking help to put a stomach-exercise program together it is certainly apparent. There are literally hundreds of exercises out there with information in bookstores, libraries and across the Internet. This can be a blessing or a curse.

With all this information how can you tell whether the exercises are any good? Listed here are a number of the most effective exercises according to recommendations by health and fitness experts.

Crunchless Crunches
Regular crunches (short sharp movements to compress your abdominal muscles) are very good for working the front part of your stomach, but do little for transverse abdominals deeper inside the midsection. While better than sit-ups, they still put strain onto your neck and back. This first exercise addresses that, working your transverse muscles more fully with less likelihood of neck or back strain.

To start, lie on your front or kneel. You may wish to try both to see which suits you to 'feel the burn' of the exercise more fully. Relax as much as you can, and try to use just the lower abdominal muscles to pull your belly button inwards toward your spine. Maintain this for at least ten seconds. If when you do this holding it for ten seconds feels too easy then build this up and hold for a slightly longer period. Then let the contraction go. Repeat this for full sets and over a relatively short time you'll start to feel the benefits.

The Hip Lift
Lie on your back on a mat or a towel then put your arms by your sides, palms facing upwards. Lift your legs so that the bottoms of your feet are pointing to the ceiling with your legs making about a ninety degree angle to your torso. Make sure that you keep your knees unbent and your legs as straight as possible. Then contract your abdominal muscles so it feels as if your navel is being pulled inward toward your spine, while at the same time gently lifting your hips off the floor. Build this up until you can raise your hips off the floor by a few inches, keeping both legs extended upward. Hold this position for a few seconds then slowly lower your hips to the floor. Repeat the exercise for a full set.

The Strong Stomach Workout

For most people setting out on any abdominal workout routine the goals are simple; either a less flabby waistline and a flatter more flattering stomach, or a stronger, more healthy set of muscles. Ideally everyone should be aiming for a balance of the two.

A flatter stomach is great and looks much more flattering, especially in a swimsuit or a pair of shorts, but in reality this is less meaningful if it is only skin deep. It is important that the central muscles as well as the outer ones are worked adequately so that the stomach area is stronger and healthier as well as more attractive. It is no use building a beautiful facade on weak foundations since beauty is only skin deep after all as the old axiom goes.

Below are a number of stomach exercises which work to create strong muscles throughout your abdomen. As with all exercise routines, be sure to take professional advice before starting and always fully warm up to prevent injury.

Toning Up Your Torso
Prepare for this exercise by kneeling on all fours, both knees and both hands flat. Still looking down, keep your stomach drawn in and extend your left arm straight out in front. Keep your arm outstretched as you extend your right leg out behind you. Bring both back to the starting position then switch your arms and legs, and repeat the exercise for a full set. Your torso and pelvis should remain static throughout.

The Butt Burner
You need to lie on your back here and we recommend using a mat or a towel. Bend your knees so that your feet remain flat to the floor with both arms by your side. Lift your pelvis and as you do so contract your buttocks so that the muscles feel squeezed tight. Raise your pelvis to forty-five degrees, so your upper body from your shoulders to your knees maintains a straight, flat ramp. Hold this for a few seconds before slowly lowering your pelvis back to the floor. Make sure that you use your stomach muscles as you lower yourself rather than letting gravity assist you. Complete an entire set of these.

The Crunchless Crunch

This exercise sounds easy but can be difficult to do well. It uses different muscles to those normally used and can be tough to get right at first. Essentially in involves contracting your stomach muscles to pull your belly button back towards your spine, compressing your stomach as you do so. You can either try this lying on your back or in a kneeling position. To start relax your body. Then slowly contract your stomach as if you are pulling your belly button backwards. Hold this for ten seconds then release slowly. Once you find ten seconds easy repeat it for longer. Building this up over time will lead to a strengthening and tightening of the transverse abdominals, one of the key interior muscle groups.

Scissor Kick

Again, lie on the floor, upper body and back tight to the ground. Place your hands under your buttocks to raise you slightly from the floor keeping your back flat. Slowly lift one leg to around ten inches and slowly (as slowly as you can manage) lower it to the floor. As you lower one leg slowly raise the other so for a short time both are in a crossing movement. Using a slow, well-controlled speed throughout is essential and will increase the effectiveness of the exercise. Repeat the exercise for a complete set.

These are only a few of the strength building exercises there are. If you are seeking to build strength across your midsection, look for exercises that work your core muscles, especially the transverse abdominals. Many components of Pilates are also excellent for this .

Using Resistance Bands In Stomach Exercises

Exercise is about working muscle groups, so exercises that do not involve resistance are unlikely to achieve very much at all, and this is particularly true with stomach and abdominal exercises. As a result, using bands can be effective as a component of any exercise routine, stomach exercises no exception.

Resistance bands are found in varying levels, often indicated by color. Green can be used where you want little resistance, yellow for medium, and red for difficult.). It is important that you choose a level which is appropriate, then move up the levels as necessary.

There is a vast number of exercises to target the stomach and abdomen that incorporate the use of resistance bands;

Seated Crunches

This exercise will provide the same basic benefits as standard crunches but with less strain without the discomfort that can come from lying on a hard surface. By using the resistance band it is this rather than gravity that provides the resistance allowing you to exercise the muscles you wish to target.

For this exercise, you need to sit in a straight backed chair. Sit straight with feet flat to the floor about hip-width apart. Contract your stomach muscles, then slowly lean forward to a 45 degree angle. You should feel the resistance from the band as you lean forward against it. Repeat this for a full set. Be sure to keep your feet to the floor, your back as straight as possible.

One-Arm Band Pulls

For this exercise stand straight with feet shoulder-width apart. Put both hands over your head with the resistance band about 18 inches apart. Then keeping your left hand over your head, move your right hand out to your side so that your elbow is bent and your hand is pointing straight up (elbow is about 90 degrees). Lower your arm until your hand is aligned with your chest then hold this position. Repeat for a full set, then switch hands.

Burning Calories: Overview

Gaining weight and losing weight are ironical to each other. One is easy to achieve and the other is quite difficult to accomplish. Increasing your calories per day is not at all a difficult task especially after a certain age.

Once you have attained a certain age, your metabolic activities reduce leading to increased weight. Young adults after a certain age complain of being overweight and desperately try to reduce their weight. This is a common occurrence nowadays and the problem has to be dealt with diligence. The solution lies in increasing your metabolic rate and the amount of calories you burn every day. The more calories you burn everyday the more weight you lose and look fit.

Most of us have the tendency to eat more with no effort on our side to reduce the amount of calories in our body. The body weight is bound to increase. We must stick to a fixed schedule of weight loss and this program should be taken very seriously and should be accorded enough significance as several other activities, which are given prime importance by us. Weight loss can be guaranteed provided our metabolic rate is increased to a certain level. Following are the suggestions for the same.

- **Movement of your body counts a lot.** The more you move the more calories you burn. Routine activities do involve a lot of movement around the house as well as in the office but the percentage should be increased to a higher level. The old maxim of moving every now and then applies true in your attempt to burn more calories.

Parking your car in the remotest corner can give your legs an exercise to reach your car. Get up in between the office hours, stretch your hands and legs, and always be in a standing position while attending the phone can distract your long period of being seated in one position and gaining weight.

- **Stimulate interest in developing muscle.** Apart from enhancing your overall personality, it also assists in burning of more calories. You are instructed to deal with weights in building muscle which goes a long way in reducing weight and gives you a fresh vibrant and young look.

Burning Calories Versus Burning Fat

Getting that perfect shape and losing weight isn't an easy task. You need to have the balance of good nutrition along with regular exercises. The foremost point that you need to understand in this is that there is a difference in burning fat and burning calories.

Our main point of focus should be on burning body fat, which is not possible by burning calories as most of us believe.

When we are exercising, it is actually the calories that we are burning, which are actually the calories within carbohydrates in our body. In order to burn calories from he fat stored in our body, there is some oxygen that is required by the body.

The method to measure this oxygen amount required by our body can be calculated by noticing the target heart rate of your body during the exercise.

Burning carbohydrates calories would mean losing water weight that decreases your metabolism. Also, carbohydrate calories that are burnt are nothing but energy calories that you are losing. Losing these calories in abundance would reduce your energy count and boost up your metabolism that buns fat indirectly.

So, you should increase your intake of calories when you are following any exercise program so that your lost energy is replaced.

Burning of fat calories at the time of exercising

There are several stages that a body goes through before reaching a point where it is actually burning the fat stored in the boy than the carbohydrates fat. Many of you must have heard people say that during your exercise, you are merely burning fat for the initial 10 minutes; it is only after that when your body asks for oxygen that you start burning the stored fat in your body.

This mark of 10 minutes can even be exceeded if you are not working very hard. Your pace while exercising should be steady, that is to say, not to slow and not to fast so that your stored fat is utilized as the source of energy.

Even if you have reached a fat burning stage doesn't mean that you will be able to maintain it as it all depends on your pace which should be right enough for you to stay there. You must be within your targeted heart rate range.

Burning of fat calories when at rest

Anaerobic exercise for weight training helps you to burn fat even after the workout. This is the key for burning fat when your body is at rest. This will help you in burning a lot of calories even more than aerobic exercise. The calories that are burnt during this time are mainly carbohydrates calories, but calories that you burn in your resting position are mostly the fat calories.

Now, because you are burning fat, when at rest id due to the fact that weight training enhances your metabolism that utilizes your stored fat in the form of energy. Last but not least, for maximum benefits, you must do both anaerobic and aerobic exercises.

Burning Calories: Keep Moving

Are you into the process of weight reduction? Move, Move and Move is the magic mantra for achieving the desired result. The increased movement of your body definitely would lead to the decrease in your weight. Dr. Wharton of Yale University has said that the more vital your exercise schedule, the more advantageous result would be achieved in regard to weight reduction.

The positive recuperating effect of the exercises on your body cannot be disputed. Due significance should be given to the fitness of your body as it solves majority of your health problems also. One has to take refuge in exercises as your companion in reducing weight. Hit the gym and face the grueling sessions of exercises mentioned in the gym for reducing weight. Set time for each activity and spend a considerable amount of time in each one of them.

For example spend about half an hour on fast walk on a walker, 20 minutes or more on aerobics, 30 minutes on route training, nearly an hour on walking alone, and several other exercises in the gym will help you in your operation of weight loss. Biking is a superb activity wherein you can burn calories to a considerable extent.

Spend some time in this activity and accomplish weight loss.

Exercises probably if done without a companion can become quite mind numbing. An acquaintance here would sort out this problem for you. Book a badminton court for playing and invite your companion to join you in the game.

Advise the companion also on the positive effects of playing the game and burning calories. All of us would want to look attractive and your incentives in this regard would definitely encourage your friend to be regular in joining you in the play.

Dancing is such a movement of the body wherein maximum amount of calories disappear from your body.

Take interest in ballroom dance, learn the dance and occasionally dance to the tunes of ballroom dance. If the right company is available with you, you can carry on the programme of weight loss even at night. A dancing session for more than 30 minutes would burn enough calories for the day.

Regular activities at home burns certain amount of calories but you can burn more if you take up activities such as cleaning the entire house, dusting the furniture, painting of the walls. Apart from the consequent weight loss, there is an additional advantage of a clean home that comes with it.

You need not venture outside the house very often for weight reduction. Choose the appropriate activities at home for a certain period of time say 45 minutes or more and that is more than enough to burn those additional calories in your body and to give you a younger and fit appearance.

Choose any one of these activities and do it on a regular basis and then accomplish a healthy and fit body that would enhance your overall personality.

Burning Calories: Aerobics

In case you are getting tired easily these days, probably you need to concentrate on getting your body in shape, build some strength in your body and count the number of calories you are consuming. Increasing strength refers to increasing the capacity of your body so that you can stand and run for more than your usual capacity, lift weights easily ad perform better in your everyday tasks.

In simple words, this will transform your body to a more enhanced version. You will not only look attractive physically like movie characters, but also able to complete your tasks without getting tired easily. All this can be achieved by aerobics exercises that need not necessarily be done at gym only. You can do them all at your home.

Aerobics exercises at home

Aerobics exercises are basically the exercises that provided the required oxygen to the body that burns calories and helps your muscles to operate in your body. Your everyday activities provided you with all the benefits of aerobic exercises, that too without wearing any of those annoying sticky Lycra uniforms.

Benefits of household aerobics exercises

Gardening and walking are the cardiovascular activities that can provide you with needed level of regular exercises. At the same time you complete your household work all by yourself such as cutting your lawn, washing you dog, shopping and others. This is also an agreed fact by all Fitness experts that aerobics exercises can help you reduce your waistline as it focuses on abdominal area where all the belly fats accumulates normally.

Just imagine, around 15 minutes of walking twice everyday can do the trick for you, that too without any dieting. Apart from the fat stored around the waistline, it helps to reduce calories and overall health of an individual.

Furthermore, people who regularly perform these household aerobics exercises also have reduced risks of suffering from cardiovascular diseases, depression, stroke, Alzheimer's disease diabetes and at times even cancer later in life.

Equation for healthy living

Hence, it is advisable to select any physical activity that you can perform regularly with interest, then select another one and gradually proceed with the task for staying healthy. This way there are fewer chances that you will quit and you will also be satisfied that you have completed so many jobs of your house.

Now if you are motivated enough to walk that extra mile for aerobics exercises, you can go for dancing, kickboxing, tai chi, swimming, gym or play tennis. The options available to you are just endless. The equation of healthy living can never be completed unless you indulge into it yourself.

Based on the above mentioned solutions, the equation can therefore be summed up as:
Aerobics + You = More Calories Burn = Increased Level of Fitness

Burning Calories: Tips For Fast Burning

With the present day generation bent more on consuming junk rather than healthy food, most people are gaining weight and growing fat these days. Though, they want to reduce their fat but they don't know how to go about it.

The main thing is to search for a reason why it happened. The reason for this is that, the number of calories that are consumed is greater in number than what has been burnt by you. So, the key lies in the fact of tuning this the other way round. That is, to increase the number of calories burnt than has been consumed.

Few tips that you can follow for this are:

1. **Build muscle** – The more the muscles, the more will be the calories that will be burnt. This is the formula that perfectly defines the idea behind this tip. You can indulge yourself in many exercises in order to build your muscle mass, but weight lifting is undoubtedly the best of all exercises to burn calories.

2. **Eat less, but frequently** – Most people generally take three meals everyday. But according to nutrition experts, consuming around five healthy meals everyday is a lot more effective to burn calories. This is because, every time you eat, your digestive system will burn food and in the process calories will also be burnt. This is an easy and great tip that can prove to be very effective to lose those extra calories.

3. **Cardio workout** – Intense cardio exercises helps you to burn more calories throughout the day than what you will burn at the time of exercising only.

4. **No need for dieting** – Diet is of no use when you are trying to burn calories. The supplement and diet industry is basically gaining from the hopes and fears of overweight people. The truth is that these alternatives may help you to reduce your water weight or muscle weight but once you stop taking them, you will gain what you have lost once again. In fact, this gain is at times more than what you were before the treatment.

Burning Calories: Treadmills

Working on treadmills is one of the best ways of exercising on machines, both to burn calories and for the ease of exercising. It has been proven in a study conducted by the VA Medical Center in Milwaukee and the Medical College of Wisconsin that calories that are burned on a treadmill are around 865-705 on an average.

Therefore, it proved to be better than stationary cycle, stair machine, rowing machine and ski machines. But, how is it possible to burn more calories in less time if you cannot take out much time for your workout?

Tips for better outcome on a treadmill

There are basically three tips given by our trainers who write for this website to super boost the calories burnt on the treadmill in lesser time:

1. **Walk uphill** – when you work on your treadmill incline, more of your muscles are made to work that burns more calories. This loss of calories can be doubled or even tripled depending upon your stamina.

But, if you cannot afford to take out 20 minutes for this workout on an incline at a stretch, you can try incline intervals. That is to say, work on a steep incline for around 1-2 minutes, and then switch for 5 minutes to the normal incline and so on.

The crux is not to allow your body to get used to a particular workout routine, which increases the amount of calories burnt even when the workout is over.

2. **Do not hold onto handrails** – Try to avoid to grip the handrails as this will reduce the efforts put on by your legs and reduce the calories burnt. As long as it is to maintain balance, it is fine.

It is better to restrict your intensity until you are not holding onto handrails for any support. It is advisable to swing your arms and carry some weight if possible, so that the whole body gets involved into it.

3. **Speed intervals** – This is similar to incline interval and increase the calories but even after the workout is over. In this, you can walk at whatever you normal pace is for around 3 minutes followed by one minute of walk at a faster pace and repeating this. This way you will definitely feel a difference in yourself after the workout.

Do not force yourself

However, make sure that you do not push yourself for such hard exercises that you start feeling aches in your body.

If you do, immediately consult a physician and slow down your pace at which you used to workout earlier.

These are the three tips that can help you burn moiré calories by investing in les time on your treadmill. It is always better t consult a doctor before starting any exercise regime.

Always be guided by the requirements of your body than what is being advised by others as everyone's body is different.

Burning Calories For Weight Loss

In case you are using the traditional aerobic cardio to lose weight, you must be spending around 30 minutes on the machine to burn certain amount of calories. It is believed that in order to lose 1 pound fat every week, you must lose 500 calories every day or every session.

This is basically a myth that people has been brain washed with. Also, whether this weight loss can be achieved through aerobic cardio is also not clear.

Calorie counting monitor installed on elliptical machines, stairmasters and treadmills is probably one of the worst inventions made ever. You may be one of those persons who have been worried by the slow pace with which the monitor creeps up at your slow cardio-sessions.

Shortcomings in the belief that losing 300-500 calories per session is necessary to lose fat

After the invention of these calorie-counting monitors, people who have been obsessed to lose around 300-500 calories every session needs to understand the loopholes in this approach.

1. **Accuracy of calorie counters** - Accuracy of calorie counters is something that cannot be commented upon as a CBS news story presented that cardio counters overestimate the calories lost by an individual by around 20%.

2. **Slow cardio inefficient for advanced loss of fat** – This is because, a study proved that men who depended only on slow cardio for weight loss, has a reduced metabolism. On the other hand, men who combined strength training with slow cardio didn't face any such problem.

Solution to lose fat

Hence, it is better to burn less calories in less time for exercising by doing interval and strength training with a little intense kind of exercising. The after burn effect will persist with this kind of exercising. For intervals, you can run for around half a minute, rest for around one minute and repeat this at least 6 times. You can use bike or treadmill if you are acquainted with it.

In these short times of intervals, the metabolic turbulence will cause a lot of calories to be burnt after the exercising so that the body is back to its normal form. Therefore, you will burn more calories and fat after exercising.

You may want to count your calories when consuming your food and it is undoubtedly important as it does make a difference. Consuming junk food would simply nullify your entire workout session of half an hour in a minute.

So, if you do not discipline yourself in terms of nutrition, even these tips would not do any good to you. Hence, interval training and keeping a check on your nutrition habits are the two methods of anti-calorie counting that helps you to reduce fat and thereby get into that perfect shape.

Burning Calories: Track The Burning

According to general fitness knowledge, it is believed that both running and walking would burn the same amount of calories every mile. However, there is no such thing that proves the truth behind this information.

Running and walking – most common exercises

Running and walking are basically two of the most common and effective ways for improving overall health and keeping up in shape of an individual. The reason for this is probably that, there is no specific training that is required for these activities to an able bodied person as opposed to activities that require correct and trained movements such as swimming, biking or swinging at the golf club.

It can be said that running and walking burns the same amount of calories considering the fact that the distance covered in both cases is the same and so should be the energy consumed in the activity. But this is not true. This is because the burning of calories is normally related to the total quantity of oxygen that is being consumed.

When you exercise continuously, you burn around five calories by consuming a liter of oxygen. Running definitely consumes more oxygen than walking, even when the distance covered is same.

More calories burnt in running than walking

A paper titled 'Energy Expenditure of Walking and Running' published in the Medicine & Science in Sports & Exercise, discussed about the study of researchers which showed the calorie burnt by 12 men and women over a distance of 1600 meters on treadmill was quite varying. While the men burnt 124 calories on an average by running, women calories burnt was counted to be 105 only.

On the other hand, while walking, the calories burnt by men amounted to 88; women figures were recorded to be 88 calories only. The calories burnt by men were more than women due to their large bodies and muscle mass.

To conclude from this, it can be said that the calorie burnt in running is around 50% more than what it used to be in walking. The reason for this disparity in calories burnt is that when a person walks, the vertical movement of gravity is quite smooth. But when a person runs, he is actually combining set of jumps together.

This leads to a constant increase and decrease in the central gravity that is affected by these jumps. Therefore, the effort or energy put in running is more than walking the similar distance.

Calculation of calories burnt

Also, what you should notice while calculating your calorie figure is the fact that there is always a difference between the net calories burnt and the total calories burnt.

Net calories are achieved by subtracting baseline calories burnt (existing calories burnt in the body) from total calories burnt. Hence, if your burn 200 calories on treadmill and your metabolism for baseline for a similar amount of time is 50 calories, your net calories would be 150 calories.

Ignoring this point, you might get mislead by an overstated calorie figure burnt by you.

Burning Calories: In Everyday Activities

Are you really interested in reducing those extra calories that too without stepping onto that exhaustive treadmill or taking laps into that swimming poll? If your answer is in the affirmative, but do not know how to do it, reading further is surely going to be of great help to you.

Burn calories by household chores

You must be shocked to know the amount of calories that you can actually reduce by doing simply household chores. This way you will not only be able to complete your household work yourself, but also be able to get back into shape by burning the extra calories that you have accumulated in your body over years.

The key lies in doing all of it briskly. If done quickly, it isn't difficult for a 150 lb person to burn up to 140 calories within half an hour of mopping the floor.

Vacuuming also burns the same amount of calories. If you iron for 30 minutes, it will also cut down 75 calories from your body.

Outdoor activities that helps to burn calories

Outdoor activities are also equally good to blow extra calories. Pulling weeds for half hour can burn 177 calories and 120 calories for tending the lawn from the same person who weighs 150 pound. Gardening often has cardiovascular and muscular benefits as it involves bending and stretching.

Car washing for one hour can take away whooping 300 calories from your body mass. Grass clipping and bagging leaves can help you burn 136 calories within half an hour.

You can even burn 130 calories if you visit a grocery store. Add another 100 calories in case you briskly walk for half an hour to reach the store. If you still fail to do all this, merely sleeping for 8 hours can help you burn 50 calories.

Indoor activities to compensate for extra calories consumed

You can easily compensate for the slice of cake that you have taken by cleaning things once the party is over. If this task takes around an hour of your efforts, you will probably end up burning 300 calories. Also, if you are in full spirit and take the initiative to wash dishes as well, you will get rid of another 152 calories. Rearranging furniture for about an hour before the party and even after it will definitely help you to do away with 450 calories more.

However, it is important to mind that all these activities should be done with great vigor and strength for maximum benefits. All this would surely be worth the cake that you had eaten.

Not to forget the home improvement activities like indoor paintings that take away 204 calories from you, installing and removing carpet and roofing that counts to 400 calories less from your body.

Nevertheless, do not forget to drink lots of water while roofing on a hot day.

Burning Calories Through Multi-Muscle Activities

Many of us are aware of the fact that resistive training helps us in building lean muscle tissue. These lean muscles then help the body in burning many calories during the training period and even when it is in the state of rest.

Hence, if you really want to burn your calories at the time of workout and even after that, you can just follow this easy guide:

1. Focus on multiple body parts - The exercises that you should choose for your training should be such that they focus upon multiple parts of the body. You can select any small or huge muscle group for this. So, rather than splitting up your entire workout, you can simply combine them into a single exercise that is also very effective.

Doing exercises such as lunge helps a person to do this effective exercise which is a combination of all and burn many calories in lesser time.

When you will perform this lunge exercise regularly you will notice a curl added to your biceps during the downward motion in lunge to acquaint the biceps, gluteals and quadriceps simultaneously. This lunge exercise is quite a dynamic exercise. This will help you to concentrate on your coordination, balance and exposure.

2. Use your fitness ball - You can also make use of a fitness ball for your dumbbell exercises. You may try to perform exercises such as shoulder and curls press and chest flies on the fitness ball, rather than merely lying and sitting on any bench.

This will definitely burn more of your calories as the unstable ball insists your body to stimulate more muscles to keep up the balance of the ball in your legs and core.

3. High intensity interval training - You can also try "high intensity interval training". This will increase your fat loss by burning more calories. Few studies done recently have proved that your metabolism can be stimulated after the workouts more than it does during the workouts by interval training than doing the training with lower intensity.

This means that even after you are over with your training still you are able to reap its benefits afterwards by burning more fats and calories for a long period of time.

However, this doesn't stand true for training with lower intensity. If you want to learn more about interval training, you can look out for Burn The Fat programs or Metabolic Surge.

So, what are you waiting for? Hurry up and make most of your time. Explore your imagination and be as creative as you can and think of all those exercises that you are presently doing and then try to change them into multi-muscle exercises.

Once you are over with this, you can gain more by your entirely new workout regime, but by giving the same amount of time.

www.ingramcontent.com/pod-product-compliance
Lightning Source LLC
Chambersburg PA
CBHW070338120526
44590CB00017B/2941